Peace With Sweets

-The Healthy & Fresh Way to Manage Sugar

Intake and Reduce Sugar Cravings-

Written by **Jordan Ring**
www.jmring.com

Peace With Sweets

Copyright © 2017 Jordan Ring
This eBook is licensed for your personal enjoyment only. This eBook may not be resold or given away to other people. If you would like to share this book with another person, please purchase an additional copy for each recipient. If you're reading this book and did not purchase it, or it was not purchased for your use only, then please return to Amazon.com and purchase your own copy. Thank you for respecting the hard work of this author.

Publishing Services Provided by

Archangel Ink

Dedication

The success of this book is a direct correlation of the efforts of my launch team. I put out feelers and 20 people jumped at the bit to sign up and help the launch of this book. You are most likely reading it because of one of these outstanding individuals.

My utmost thanks to them:

-Brian Goldman (Running Without Injuries Blog), Karen Wiedmeier, Pamela Sloss, Mike Karnes, Michael Ring, Alicia Veenstra, Jessica Massaway, Laura Ostrem, Nate Johnson, Marsha Irvin, Tom Miner, Anita Warren, Enzi Alexander Jauregui, Travis Stephenson, Kimbre Varney, Sean Chase, Pamela Gardner, Darlene Holley, Melinda Ring, Cameron Browning.

Disclaimer

The information contained in this guide is for informational purposes only. I'm not a lawyer or an accountant. Any legal, financial, fitness, or weight loss advice that I give is my opinion based on my own experience. You should always seek the advice of a professional before acting on something that I have published or recommended.

Publication of any such Third Party Material is simply a recommendation and an expression of my own opinion of that material. No part of this publication shall be reproduced, transmitted, or sold in whole or in part in any form, without the prior written consent of the author. All trademarks and registered trademarks appearing in this guide are the property of their respective owners.

Users of this guide are advised to do their own due diligence when it comes to making personal decisions and all information, products, services that have been provided should be independently verified by your own qualified professionals. By reading this guide, you agree that myself and my company is not responsible for the success or failure of your personal decisions relating to any information presented in this guide.

Your Free Bonus

See below for an awesome bonus related to the super awesome content in this book. I promise it won't contain excessive use of the word awesome.

You can choose to sign up for my email list if you want on my site's home page, or go to my book's resources page to download them all with no strings attached.

Http://www.jmring.com

Included in the bonus:

1. Sample personal blueprint
2. PDF of the sugary foods to avoid
3. PDF of the common foods to eat

Table of Contents

Part One: Why Am I Reading This Book?

Chapter One: Soda is Like a Cheat Code......................**6**
Chapter Two: Sugar's Deepest, Darkest Secrets On Display..**10**
Chapter Three: The Anatomy of a Sugar Beast............**22**
Chapter Four: The Urge to Eat Dessert:
Sugar Addiction..**28**

Part Two: Taking Action to Reduce Sugar Intake

Chapter Five: Be Mindful Young Padawan..................**36**
Chapter Six: Choosing the Right Foods.......................**45**
Chapter Seven: Prep the Battleground..........................**52**
Chapter Eight: Exercise as a Means Of Reducing Cravings..**60**
Chapter Nine: Build Your Personal Blueprint..............**65**
Chapter Ten: Consistency Through Course
Adjustments..**75**
Final Thoughts and a Kick in the Butt..........................**79**
A Quick Favor Please?..**81**
About the Author..**82**

Why Am I Reading This Book?

Part One

> *"Change will not come if we wait for some other person or some other time. We are the ones we've been waiting for. We are the change that we seek." - Barack Obama*

Let's get down to brass tacks. Drop that sour gummy worm and read this: You can beat your sugar addiction.

You are reading this book because you probably need to nix your obsession with frozen cow's milk. At the very least you want to reduce sugar cravings so you can finally eat a meal without the immediate firing of "holy cow I need a milkshake" from your brain neurons.

Sweet and sugary drinks, mounds of cake, and the sneaky "health food" options that we are constantly shoving in our faces make our relationship with sugar less than peaceful. In fact, for most of us there is no way to feel good about eating a piece of chocolate cake.

Let me take a wild guess: You love the taste of chocolate? Especially a sweet velvety piece of cake? How about a candy bar, or a scrumptious bag of chocolate-covered pretzels?

How hard it is to constantly wrestle with these thoughts, and how often are we actually able to resist? Believe me, I know how hard it is to resist even one candy bar, but when we have to say no for 3, 4, or even 7 days straight? Forget about it. This is where most of us fail and then struggle to continue living healthy.

This book will lessen the effect these urges have on you by empowering you to make better decisions, arm you with the knowledge of where to find added sugar, and give you the practical tools necessary to win the battle against the sugar beast. Making peace with sweets is not something you can do in one day. The good news is that it's definitely doable over time, and learning how to win the small battles will increase your overall health resiliency.

There are many different factors and tactics to consider when trying to lose weight and live healthy. I outline many of these tactics in my book "The Action Diet."

The Action Diet is designed to show you small changes that you can group together in order to achieve your weight loss goals.

One of those tactics was to reduce sugar intake. In that book I just scratched the surface of the benefits of reducing sugar intake, but I realized afterwards that sugar is a subject people would like to know more about, especially when it comes to how to stop eating so freaking much of it.

This book is going to take an in-depth look at sugar and answer the following questions:

1. Why is sugar the enemy?
2. Why is sugar so addicting?
3. What do I do if I love drinking soda or other sweet drinks?
4. What steps can I take to find peace with sweets?

After reading this book you'll have tactics that will make it possible to eat a piece of cake without feeling the gut-wrenching pang of guilt when that last bite goes from the fork to your mouth. You'll also be able to say no to your mom's homemade mint brownies without feeling guilty.

This book will serve as a wake up call to get you on the right path and also be a fun guide to learning about sugar.

Merriam-Webster defines "peace" as- "a state of tranquility or quiet."

The key is to come to a state of peace with the foods you are putting into your body, regardless of how healthy that food might be. It is true that you cannot find peace by having 3 cans of soda every day, but if you limit your intake or replace it with a suitable alternative, you can indeed have peace with your decision.

The chapters in this book will arm you for the battle that you have to wage within in order to reach a state of tranquility with each dietary decision you make. Each and every day you will be tested. Life will continue to throw down the gauntlet at your feet day after day and you need to be prepared.

Making peace with sweets is something you must fully give yourself to. A half-hearted attempt to vanquish the sugar beast will leave you worse off than before.

Gear up and let me show you how to win the war against sugar so you can lose weight and live the healthy life you deserve.

Are you ready for a sweet battle?

Let's go.

Chapter One: Soda is Like a Cheat Code

In J.R.R. Tolkien's The Lord of the Rings trilogy, the Dead Men of Dunharrow, an army of ghosts, was utilized by the king of Gondor to defeat the minions of Mordor. The green mass swept through the battlements and destroyed everything in its path. These undead warriors could not be killed, stopped, or even hurt whatsoever.

In the Peter Jackson movie adaptations, using this army of the dead was basically a cheat code to guarantee a win. It gave the orcs, trolls, and mercenaries no chance and it wasn't fair. Check out this Youtube video (http://bit.ly/2nHv8UJ) for a quick view of the destruction they can wreak.

Not that any of us were rooting for the orcs anyways, but this army was deadly in its use and execution. It invaded the enemy and overtook them like a wave over rocks.

Fortunately for the Dark Lord Sauron, this cheat code was a one-time use and it could not then be turned on him at the Black Gates.

Unfortunately for you, sugar is ever present and can be used against you at any time. Sugar is one badass cheat code used to make you fat, deplete your energy, and cause disease.

Sugar is an army of the dead for your body, and while your immune system is much stronger than a mere orc, your chances of fighting off the invasion forever are quite slim.

Imagine the Army of the Dead pouring down your gullet. With each sip you are pumping in a calvary of liquid sugar intent on wreaking chaos on your system. Every single time you drink a bottle of Mountain Dew, three things happen to your body within one hour:

First 30 Minutes

Your system is hit with an overwhelming amount of sugar all at once. Actually, one bottle of mountain dew has TWICE the amount of sugar men should have per day and THREE times as much for women.

According to the American Heart Association, men should take in no more than 150 calories of sugar per day (37.5 grams or 9 teaspoons). Women should take in no more than 100 calories per day (25 grams or 6 teaspoons).

One bottle of mountain dew simply is too much for your system to handle once, let alone on a regular basis.

45 Minutes

Blood sugar spikes and your liver goes into overdrive, turning any available sugar into fat. The liver doesn't know what to do with all the invaders and it throws the sugar into storage bin under the bed (fat cells).

The great news is that our bodies are built like fortresses and are incredibly resilient. However, even Helm's Deep was overtaken by a consistent press. Once we drink soda and eat sweets too many times, our bodies begin to wear out. The resulting problem is insulin resistance, which I will discuss in depth later on in this book.

One Hour

Caffeine has finished its path through your body and has been fully absorbed. Your pupils dilate, blood pressure rises, and dopamine production goes up, which stimulates the pleasure centers of your brain.

At this point you feel great. The caffeine is working and the sugar has given you a happy feeling that is spreading to your toes. Don't get too excited; this feeling won't last and is NOT good for your body. But you got this far might as well enjoy the feeling. Go ahead, dance around, be crazy, and laugh like a madman.

The After Effects

The diuretic properties of soda have caused a quick trip to the bathroom. The caffeine boost has hit a high, but you know you will be coming down soon with a severe afternoon crash.

Either your head is hitting your desk, or you are forced to drink a second bottle to stay productive. The cycle of sugar-boosted energy has begun and you feel stuck in its deadly grasp.

This is the process of allowing the Army of the Dead to enter into your system. It is like a cheat code for the enemy because it tastes so damn good, but it is so freaking bad for you.

Cupcakes, chocolate-covered pretzels, and fruit juices have similar effects to that of soda, but are admittedly not as bad for you because they at least have one redeeming quality. Soda has none whatsoever.

For this reason, the very first step in finding peace with sweets is to reduce your soda intake severely or limit it completely. There is no peace of mind when it comes to drinking soda, because there is absolutely nothing good going for you when you drink it.

Stop letting the enemy use its favorite cheat code. Limit soda intake and never again fear the Army of the Dead.

Chapter Two: Sugar's Deepest, Darkest Secrets On Display

Sugar deserves to be taken apart with every sneaky little granular on display for the world to see. Knowing what sugar truly is and how it can affect your body can go a long in helping you to become more aware of it, since many food companies try to hide it in different foods.

This chapter will give a quick and simple rundown of the different parts of sugar and how they all work together.

You can't have peace with sweets if you are ignorant to how pervasive sugar has become in our diet.

Secret One: Not all Sugar is Bad

The good news? Some forms of sugar are not as bad as they seem. It shouldn't be surprising that apples are good for you, despite claims that you should limit fruit intake in order to reduce sugar intake. What kind of advice is that!? Hey look there is an apple that grew naturally from a tree, probably shouldn't eat it because it contains sugar.

It's not that simple. Sugar in some capacity is necessary for energy and our survival, but if not treated with respect, it can be our undoing.

Not all sugar is created equal.

Secret Two: What is Sugar?

The two most common forms of sugar are fructose and glucose, but all sugar is a carbohydrate that our bodies break down and use for energy. Chances are that if it ends in "ose," it' a sugar.

Not to go too Bill Nye here, but each type of naturally-occurring sugar falls into a different grouping of either monosaccharides or disaccharides. Put simply, monosaccharides are simple sugars that cannot be broken down further. Disaccharides are made up of two simple sugars put together by glycosidic linkage.

Don't worry, it's not much more complicated! Here are the different kinds of naturally-occurring sugar that we need to be concerned with (We will get to sugar substitutes later):

Fructose appears in cane sugar and honey, but most often in fruits. Fructose is broken down by your liver and doesn't initiate a response by insulin.

Glucose is another natural form of sugar that our bodies can produce on its own if needed. It is either burned as energy or turned into glycogen for use later on. Glucose can be found naturally in fruits and plants. Glucose breaks down in the stomach and thus insulin is released into the bloodstream to metabolize the glucose completely.

Sucrose (also known as table sugar) can be found in the stems of sugarcane or the roots of sugar beet. Sucrose is broken down into fructose and glucose during digestion.

Lactose is a milk sugar and the reason some people can't drink milk. If you have any lactose-intolerant friends you are well aware of this phenomenon. Some people are unable to drink milk or eat ice cream without a fast trip to the bathroom.

These naturally-occurring sugars can also be processed and made into the white table sugar that we eat each and every day.

At this point it is worth talking about the difference between real and added sugar.

Secret Three: The Difference Between Real and Added Sugar

Natural vs. unnatural is not enough of a distinction to determine the main difference between real and added sugars.

The difference is the act of what is done to the food. Taking a spoonful of sugar to make the medicine go down is an act of adding sugar.

Eating a freshly plucked apple off a tree is an act of eating real sugar. One medium apple contains 19 grams of sugar, which might surprise you. However, that sugar is mostly fructose, with some glucose and sucrose present as well.

Remember that fructose is broken down by the liver and the blood sugar spike is usually not substantial. Better yet, there is virtually no limit to how much natural sugar you can eat per day according to the FDA.

Apples also contain important vitamins and minerals, as well as a lot of fiber. Fiber slows down the absorption of the sugar before it finds its way into the liver. YES! Fiber wins again!

If you cut up your apple, remove the skin, and dip it in caramel, you are adding a ton of sugar (and of course, removing the skin reduces the fiber content significantly). Yes the sugar found in the apple is natural, but altering the taste in order to enjoy it more fully is the definition of added sugars.

Real sugar is found in the natural form of fruits, vegetables, and dairy products with nothing done to alter the sweetness.

Added sugars are any type of sugar that is purposely added or sneaked into food in order to alter the taste.

Eating real sugar is okay, and even encouraged. Eating too much added sugar is bad and should be avoided at all costs.

Eat fruits and vegetables daily. Give your body the real energy that it needs in order to function. Avoid added sugars by limiting intake of processed foods.

Secret Four: Glycemic Index and Glycemic Load Unpacked.

You have probably heard of the glycemic index, but you may be ignorant to what it actually means.

The glycemic index was created by Dr. David Jenkins, a professor of nutrition at the University of Toronto, in 1981. It's a system that assigns point values to foods based on how slowly or quickly those foods cause increases in blood glucose levels (blood sugar). A low point value means that the glucose is released slowly and steadily over time. A high point value means that the glucose is rapidly introduced.

You might be making the confused face at me again, but bear with me. The glycemic index is important because awareness of the processes our bodies are undertaking after eating a candy bar is essential to winning the war against sugar.

To get the complete picture of how a food will affect your system, you need to know how quickly the food makes glucose enter the bloodstream, and how much glucose it will deliver. This determination is called the glycemic load (GL).

The glycemic load is figured out by multiplying the grams of carbohydrate in a serving by the glycemic index of the specific food, then dividing by 100. This gives a more accurate picture of the process as a whole because the level of carbohydrate in a food is factored in.

Anything ten or below is good. Eleven to nineteen is average. Twenty or above is considered high.

Here are a few foods with their glycemic load indicated:

All Bran (cereal)- 4
Orange- 4
Milk Full-Fat- 5
Apple- 5
Baked Beans- 6
Banana- 16
Cornflakes- 19
Brown Rice- 21
Linguine- 21
Bagel- 24

(For a more comprehensive list, click here (http://bit.ly/1tTTpDB), or see this chart (http://bit.ly/2nfNkd3.)

This table is just a quick look at different types of foods. Again, you can see that fruits are in the low to medium range on the scale, while breads and pastas are higher.

Unless you need a major boost for an intense workout or a long-distance run, familiarize yourself with low GL foods and eat a diet that consists mostly of them. I will give a much more comprehensive action plan in the coming chapters, along with lists of the right foods to eat and ones to avoid.

Think twice before you combine a bagel with a banana and put yourself in the glycemic hole by breakfast. This will only lead to falling over the ledge later on when you eat a piece of cake, and when you feel sick afterwards you will know why.

The bottom line? Stick with food items that have a low glycemic load in order to reverse and prevent the effects of a high sugar diet.

Secret 5: Tricky Added Sugar Names

One more dirty secret that sugar is loathe to share is that it has many aliases. It goes by so many names it is almost impossible to remember them all.

Here are the five I believe are most prevalent but you can see this infographic (http://bit.ly/2o66TD4) that shares 60 different names for sugar.

High-fructose corn syrup
Agave nectar
Evaporated cane juice
Corn sweetener
Dextrose

There is no need to memorize these or any of the other 60 names for sugar. Instead, be mindful of the most common foods you are eating. I once discovered that a Kellogg's "fiber bar" that I was eating every day for over a year was actually high in trans fats, sugar of all kinds, and scored poorly on the Fooducate App.

It pays to be aware and to check the labels of every food you eat, but you definitely need to check the contents of the foods you eat the most.

Take a large chocolate shake from McDonalds for example. It has 840 calories, 109 grams of carbs, 119 grams of sugar, and countless other sugar ingredients listed...

But it tastes so freaking good!

Thus the struggle, and thus the reason why you cannot be ignorant any longer. You can't have peace with your decision to order a large chocolate shake at the drive-thru unless you understand what you are imparting to your body.

You might think that ignorance is bliss, and in the case of a milkshake it's hard to argue that. But I think it is possible to be able to enjoy a milkshake AND also understand that you might want to wait a while before that next trip to the drive-thru.

Secret 6: Sugar Substitutes: A Good Alternative?

There are several different types of sugar alternatives. I've broken them down into three groups: Won't Upset the Sugar Beast, Stay Far Away, and On The Fence.

Won't Upset the Sugar Beast

I am labeling these as acceptable replacements to sugar because they have SOME redeeming qualities. I think it's good to have a balanced diet, and if you absolutely have to sweeten up your food, it is better to do it with something that will add some nutritional value to your daily intake.

1) Honey: An acceptable alternative to sugar in small quantities. It would be best to get it locally, but I have read conflicting research about whether or not that makes a difference. I like honey because among other health benefits, it is a natural decongestant. This is fantastic for anyone that struggles with allergies like I do.

Important to note here is the difference between raw

honey and processed golden honey. If you are looking to get more benefits and avoid unwanted side effects, choose the raw variety.

Too much of anything can be a bad thing, and at the end of the day honey is still made of mostly fructose. Adding a little bit of honey to your tea won't hurt anything, just be cautious of how much you are using by keeping in mind that it still counts as added sugar.

2) Maple syrup: I know what you are picturing: a stack of pancakes with a boat load of syrup on them. Man that is a tasty image, I apologize for making you want to stop reading in order to cook up a few right now! Anyways, maple syrup has been shown to contain antioxidants that can be a useful addition to our immune system.

And we are all probably guilty of doing this, but don't pour a boatload on your pancakes by "accident" and then feel obliged to eat them anyways. As with all things balance is key, no need to drown your pancakes.

3) Molasses: It's packed full of minerals and is even a good source of iron. It is high in fructose, but again, it has a redeeming quality so it qualifies as acceptable, but only in small doses.

If you are going for something sweet can't find a better alternative, look to molasses.

4) Xylitol: Often found in chewing gum because of its ability to prevent tooth decay and cavities, xylitol is a sugar alcohol found in plant material. It's also a medicine that is used to prevent middle ear infections in children. Xylitol has fewer calories than sugar, and with a glycemic index of only 7, it doesn't raise blood sugar levels.

As far as picking a pack of gum is concerned, xylitol is safe--just don't add an abundance to your coffee.

Stay Far Away

Scrambling to protect their image and to provide every single person with an option that meets their dietary requirements, food companies have resorted to natural and lab-created alternatives to sugar.

The effects of these alternative options are mostly unresearched and yet they are still being paraded as the safer alternative option. This is extreme for me to say, but don't fall for these lies. If it sounds too good to be true it probably is.

For me, I never liked the taste of diet soda or diet anything for that matter. I drank soda knowing full well that it was bad for me. Obviously, this approach was bad too, but I never developed a tolerance for fake sugar. Instead, I could always taste it because I knew right away if the food I was eating contained aspartame or another alternative. I know some that like the taste and that is fine, just be careful of being the guinea pig for an under researched alternative.

1) High Fructose Corn Syrup: This one is just bad, bad, bad. There is nothing redeeming about HFCS, and it's ridiculously prevalent in the American diet.

HFCS is made from refining corn into a mixture of glucose and fructose. Since it is so cheap to make compared to any other type of sugar, it is used as a sweetener in almost all processed foods.

This makes it extremely dangerous because it is so hard to avoid. If you have ever had to cook for someone that is both gluten and dairy free, you understand how much foods in the grocery store have in common. Trying to shop and go completely sugar free is another story altogether.

HFCS can be found in sweet drinks, so-called "health foods," and even crackers. If you see this on the label it is a good sign that you might want to put the food back and find something else.

Definitely avoid this at all costs.

2) Agave Syrup: This is a syrup that is made from the Agave tequilana (tequila) plant and is actually about 1 1/2 times sweeter than regular sugar. While agave sounds natural, it's still not a good option, as it has a higher fructose content than normal sugar with zero redeeming qualities.

3) Brown Rice Syrup: This syrup has a higher glycemic index (97) than normal sugar (68) and even pure glucose (96). It also could potentially contain arsenic. Avoid at all costs.

4) Aspartame: Also known as Equal, NutraSweet and Spoonful, aspartame is definitely on the list of sugar alternatives to avoid. Aspartame has been linked to cancer, obesity, diabetes, headaches, blindness, brain tumors, seizures, Alzheimer's and Parkinson's disease, and other neurological disorders in multiple studies.

Just like we wouldn't want to replace a broken washing machine with a broken washboard, there is no good reason to reach for a sugar alternative that causes more harm than sugar itself.

5) Sucralose: Also known as Splenda, sucralose is created from table sugar when 3 hydrogen-oxygen groups are replaced with chlorine atoms. Picture a swimming pool filled with sugar and then the resulting gunk is scooped up into little yellow packets for everyday use.

Sucralose has been shown to be safe in some studies, but in others shows it might affect our gut bacteria, raise blood sugar and insulin levels, and may not be safe to cook with due to the fact that at temperatures above 350 harmful substances may be formed.

On The Fence

These sugar alternatives have not seen enough research to have decisive conclusions about their safety. If you are utilizing any of these alternatives, be aware that it is unknown what they are doing to your body.

The following sugar alternatives are relatively new to the scene. When aspartame was first introduced, I'm sure it was heralded as the great savior to the junk food industry, but look at it now. The propensity for big corporations to push "healthy" new sugar alternatives without adequate research is as present now as it ever was.

Realistically, the junk food and soda industry could potentially research and introduce a new sugar substitute much faster than anyone in authority could do anything about. It would get out on the market, be touted as extremely healthy and safe, and then years later research might get out that it causes cancer or another serious illness.

The next thing you know these companies ditch this alternative in order to find a new one and repeat the process all over again. This is is why I am on the fence with the following alternatives. I just don't trust that their creators have our best interests at heart.

1) Stevia: Stevia is a plant native to South America. The leaves are used as sweetener. The problem with utilizing stevia as a sweetener is getting it in its natural form. It its refined state it can be just as bad as other sugar substitutes because it might be mixed with unknown ingredients.

Truvia is the sugar brand most associated with stevia, but it only contains certain ingredients from the plant, along with many other additives. It's also, you guessed it, highly processed!

I recommend avoiding stevia until further research is conducted, but if you want to give it a try, make sure you are getting the natural stevia leaves with nothing extra added.

2) Monk Fruit Sweetener: A natural zero calorie sweetener that is extracted from the monk fruit that grows in southeast Asia, where it is very popular. It's been used for many years in that region as a sugar substitute that is over 100 times sweeter than actual sugar. The research is still out as to its healthiness, but is very promising.

If you feel inclined to try it, be sure to read the label and get only monk fruit without any additives.

3) Coconut Palm Sugar: This sugar substitute contains the minerals Iron, Zinc, Calcium and Potassium. Coconut sugar is made by cutting the flower of the coconut palm and extracting the liquid sap into containers. The sap is then placed under heat until most of the water has evaporated.

Made in this way, this type of sugar retains some of its nutrients which makes it healthier than either regular sugar or HFCS.

I've added it to the on the fence section because it is still loaded with fructose, and any of the possible health benefits from the nutrients are outweighed by this.

At the end of the day, any sugar substitute is still an act of adding sugar. You need to focus on reducing the need to add sugar to anything and everything you eat, and instead eat natural fruits and veggies.

As far as liquid nourishment goes, drinking water is king. Every single time you choose it instead of another drink you are doing yourself a huge favor.

There is no sugar substitute that can take the place of eating a balanced diet, and the more that you focus on eating healthy foods, the less you will have the need to replace sugar with a sugar substitute.

Chapter Three: The Anatomy of a Sugar Beast

Now that we have the dirty secrets out of the way, let's delve into why sugar is so bad for us and why I call it the sugar beast (hint: it isn't fluffy, isn't nice, and doesn't want to dance with the lady in the castle).

In this chapter I'm only talking about the sugar that's added to foods. Soda, candy, some bread, sweet tea, etc. are all culprits here.

The army of the dead is a cheat code that sugar uses in the form of soda, but consistent intake is equivalent to unleashing every orc and goblin from within Mordor itself.

If you keep ingesting too much sugar the following things could happen to you. If you already deal with some of these issues, don't sweat it, because everyone starts somewhere. We will learn how to beat down the sugar beast in further chapters!

It Makes You Fat From Insulin Resistance

Insulin is a hormone produced by your pancreas that allows glucose to be used for energy. Every time you ingest sugar that contains glucose, your body will release insulin to burn the glucose for energy or store it as glycogen in your muscles or liver.

This is a completely normal process. Where it gets complicated and starts to change things for the worse is when we introduce either high levels of fructose or high levels of glucose over time. This will eventually lead to prediabetes and then full blown type two diabetes.

Ingesting high levels of glucose over time cause the insulin that's released to be less effective and have to work harder.

Think of it like the Death Star. Your body is the Death Star, while the Rebel Alliance is sugar. As the Death Star, your body releases tie fighters (insulin) to fight off the invaders. For a while the Rebel Alliance is held off and the Empire is winning.

But then the Rebel Alliance pushes back. Eventually they get through a weak point and blast the Death Star to smithereens.

The analogy stops working there because your body isn't going to explode. But if you continue to allow the Rebel Alliance to beat down your body eventually you will become insulin resistance, get prediabetes, and be at risk for getting type two diabetes.

Constant high levels of insulin cause glucose to be stored in our fat cells readily and often. This fat is often hard to get to because the body gets confused and doesn't tap into this source of energy, instead opting to tell us to eat more food.

High levels of fructose are even worse for our system, causing insulin resistance by overwhelming the liver, leading to nonalcoholic fatty liver disease. The disease will then in turn into hepatic insulin resistance, which will eventually lead to type two diabetes.

Glucose is normal for our bodies to deal with, but too much of it can be a bad thing. Fructose is nothing our bodies can't handle in low amounts, such as what you would get from fruits, but added sugar contains a ton and overwhelms our system.

Added sugar is the killer.

Insulin resistance is just the beginning effect of eating too much sugar. The next step is prediabetes, which means that your blood sugar level is higher than it should be. People that currently have prediabetes are very likely to develop type two diabetes if their lifestyles go unchanged.

The best way to see where you currently fall on this continuum is get checked out by a doctor. If that isn't an option, then reducing sugar intake and seeing how you feel is a good first step. If you get a major crash right away from not having a soda with lunch then it might be time to make a long-term, consistent change.

Just remember that it isn't too late for anyone to get on the right path. Hang tight and this book will lead you there. You might even enjoy the process.

Sugar's effect on leptin

Leptin is a hormone secreted by fat cells that regulates our appetite by sending signals to our brain. When working properly, increased leptin production means that we don't eat as much because we feel full.

Leptin: "Hey you! Stop eating!"

You: "Oh okay, you're right. I am full! I'll stop now."

But once a body becomes leptin resistant, the conversation changes.

Leptin: "Hey I'm getting really full here! Seriously, stop eating!"

You: "I could probably eat at least one more plate of spaghetti… muahaha...ONE!? Try two!"

Leptin helps to regulate and keep our bodies in a constant state of energy balance, not swinging too far either way.

Leptin resistance is just part of the problem that a high sugar diet causes. It is part of the downward journey that anyone that eats too much sugar experiences. It's not surprising that millions of people struggle with the effects of not feeling full after eating more than enough to meet their basic needs.

Cortisol

Cortisol is also known as the stress hormone. It's important that we know what it is and how sugar can affect it, because most of us are stressed in some fashion, whether it be from a crazy job, a newborn at home, or money issues.

Here is how this hormone is supposed to work:

1. A bear pops out of the woods while you're on a hike.
2. Cortisol is blasted into your body, which in turn floods your muscles with glucose.
3. You are faced with the fight or flight response; your body has been primed to do whichever one

is more likely to result in your survival.
4. Insulin production is limited in order to burn glucose instead of storing it.
5. Arteries are narrowed, increasing heart rate.
6. You either fight the bear and lose, run away, or back away slowly, but the rush of adrenaline is enough to do what needs to be done.
7. Everything returns to normal once you're safe (unless you died from the bear attack… sorry...)

This entire process is normal for us to experience every once in awhile. However, within the stressful lifestyle that most of us live in, we face it almost constantly.

Just the other day I had this experience at work, where I'm a manager at a retirement community. I was walking around pouring coffee for our residents. I was hit with a lot at once. I was asked to get more creamer, grab some water, and then I realized that we had to serve over 100 people, needed to make more coffee, AND I had to answer the phone.

I felt the fight or flight response keenly. I wanted to hightail it out of the dining room. But I had to stay. I could feel the rush of overwhelm that comes along with too many people asking too much of you.

Consistent stress and high levels of cortisol can effectively render you insulin resistant without even adding sugar intake on top of that.

When this process happens too often in our bodies, things start to break down. When we add a high sugar diet to a stressful lifestyle things can go haywire. Our bodies end up starved of glucose, sending stress signals to the brain.

We then eat more sugar to help out, but because we are stressed this sugar does not not get stored as glycogen. It's one nasty cycle that can be really hard to break.

It is a marriage made in the pits of hell because either one can be bad, but together they wreak havoc on your system.

Feeding the unhealthy bacteria

There is now plenty of research (http://bit.ly/1FjkZlb) that shows how sugar can affect our bodies as well as our minds, specifically our ability for cognitive flexibility (adapting to new stimuli). Interestingly enough, the root problem seems to be within our gut.

Some scientists are even calling Alzheimer's disease type 3 diabetes, due to the growing evidence that sugar consumption plays a major role in our brains.

Sugar alternatives are just as much to blame here, and research suggests that consuming too much can alter the system of healthy bacteria in your gut by promoting the growth of the "bad" bacteria and preventing the growth of "good" bacteria.

I've seen the effect that dementia can have on folks first hand in the retirement community. It breaks my heart when Katherine, a resident who's lived at the community for months introduces herself to me every single day. I just smile and nod and tell her that I know her name, but that I am so happy that she is here with us.

There isn't much more you can do in these scenarios other than smile and move on, but it scares me. Is there a day that my mom or dad might not recognize me? The potential pain is too great to ignore.

I hope I never have to introduce myself to my own parent, and I hope the same for you.

If potentially having issues related to dementia later on in life isn't enough of a reason to reduce sugar intake, I'm not sure what is.

Sugar is bad for so many reasons, even beyond weight control.

Are you convinced yet?

Chapter Four:
The Urge to Eat Dessert: Sugar Addiction

Chances are you might be addicted to sugar if you feel an overwhelming craving to order dessert after finishing up your first three courses. Lets face it, does anyone ever "save room" for dessert? Isn't there ALWAYS room for dessert?

Most of us that eat sugar on a regular basis are actually addicted. Sugar induces addiction in much the same way as alcohol, cannabis, tobacco, and cocaine. All of these substances affect the pleasure center of the brain (the nucleus accumbens) by making you want more and more of it.

Eventually, you get so much of it that it stops making you feel "good' instead acting as a means to keeping you at a stationary level. It is at this point that it becomes an addiction, in that if you stopped partaking in sugary foods you will readily feel the effects of withdrawal.

If you are in the mood for a quick video, check out this one (http://bit.ly/1lCsdtm) on just how addicting sugar is.

In short it explains the process in which we become addicted to sugar:

1. We eat sugar
2. Dopamine is released into the pleasure center in the brain
3. We continue to eat sugar in high doses
4. Dopamine receptors are overwhelmed
5. The next time we eat more sugar the effects are blunted, causing us to want to eat more sugar.

Does any of this sound familiar?

Are you craving your next meal or the dessert after the meal?

Do you add sugar to every food you eat?

Would it be hard for you to quit sugar for one full day?

If you answered yes to any of these questions, then there's a good chance you might be addicted. I don't think we need to fear the word addiction or think less of ourselves if we are addicted, because facing the truth is often the first step towards enlightenment and progress.

We also need to decide if the addiction is something we want to act upon. I am personally addicted to coffee as I am usually planning out how I will get to my coffee in the morning, and at what point in the afternoon I would like another cup. I don't believe that drinking coffee in moderate amounts is bad for me, but I would also say that I am addicted because going one or two days without it would severely limit my level of functioning.

But with coffee I don't really want to break the addiction.

When it comes to sugar, I definitely do want to break the addiction. Right now I still have more sugar than I need. I have done away with drinking a soda every day, and I never add sugar to my coffee, but there are many other mistakes I make.

If I would have to hazard a guess I would say that you are in a similar situation with your sugar cravings. Your brain feels hijacked and you immediately crave dessert after almost every single meal. Your mouth even starts to salivate, even when you know that you

A) don't need it and
B) really don't need it.

The good news is that being addicted to sugar is not something you did on purpose. You probably wouldn't even wish the addiction on your worst enemy, unless of course that enemy was Darth Vader, then I would say throw the cake, pray, and get the heck out of there!

The bad news is that you have to make the change, no one else can do it for you. You are an amazing person with the potential to move mountains, but you have to be willing to start somewhere in order to tap into that potential.

I don't know is how fate decided to act in your life. I don't know whether or not you grew up on chicken nuggets and french fries loaded in ketchup, were given M&Ms as a reward for good behavior, or still count on a sugary treat to help with a miserable day.

But none of that is a good enough excuse to not take a step in the right direction. What I do know is that you can start today strong.

For the purposes of this book, you need to first recognize that only you have the power to change and fend off the forces of evil. Defeating the sugar beast and finding peace with sweets starts with your willingness to fight back, suffer a little bit, and then become victorious.

Sugar addiction can be beaten. You can choose to eat a slice of cake without then having to find the source of the slice and finishing off the entire monstrosity. You do not need to live in fear that you will again slip up with your diet and break down completely.

Like any addiction, breaking your habit of eating sugar with every meal is not going to be easy. The very first time you resist, you'll feel the effects strongly. You're fighting against your brain for control. It is almost like a real life sugar beast is inside your brain telling you whatever it can to get you to get that next fix.

Have you ever told yourself or a friend:

"Wow great job not eating that cupcake, you definitely deserve to eat a large piece of pie later."

"What's wrong with taking just a small bite?" Then BAM, the entire Milky Way is gone.

"Wanna share a dessert? We deserve it!"

We are fighting against ourselves in order to break the addiction and get on solid ground. On the one hand we can see the light and our brains want to help us out, but the feeling of dopamine being released is like a master masseuse rubbing her hands all over the insides of your mind. The feeling is just too great to avoid sometimes.

Taking action on advice is the single most difficult part about making a change in your life. I believe most books only give a passing effort to tell you how you should do whatever it is they are suggesting is important.

My approach is quite different. I spend more time in the practical, because this is more important in the long run.

Taking Action to Reduce Sugar Intake

Part Two

"Action is the foundational key to all success."
-Pablo Picasso

There is no single entity that exists more capable of making change than you and your very own two feet (and your hands--drop that donut you just grabbed). The only way to lose weight, eat healthier, and live longer is to make a change to your lifestyle.

This section will guide you towards the action steps necessary to reduce your sugar intake and to find the peace with sweets that you have always dreamed of. Each section will give concrete examples of how to do it.

Taking action to reduce sugar intake includes the following steps.

1. **Recognize**- Understand what it is you are putting into your body.
2. **Eat Low Sugar Foods**- Find other foods you can eat that have less sugar but still taste good.
3. **Alter your environment**- The old maxim of "out of sight, out of mind" is as true today as when John Heywood first wrote it in 1562.
4. **Exercise**- Outlines the benefits of exercise relating to sugar intake and how to get started.
5. **Taking Ownership**- Build your own personal blueprint and become accountable for your choices.
6. **Readjust course and stay consistent**- There will always come a time when you start to slack off, and you will need to reevaluate your current status and start fresh.

The Following chapters will dicuss these six steps in greater detail. You will learn that taking action is doable as long as you maintain consistency.

It is only by mastering these steps that you'll learn to become one with the force and reduce your sugar intake.

Chapter Five: Be Mindful Young Padawan

One cool part of the Star Wars saga was when Qui Gon Jin yelled "Duck Anakin!" in the Phantom of the Menace.

Anakin, who was only 9 years old at the time, immediately and without a word of protest or even a questioning glance, ducked and narrowly avoided a speeder bike implanted into his back. Yes, of course, the force was on his side, but he was aware enough and trusting enough to follow his new master's directions.

Recognizing your current situation is the very first step in meeting any goal, but is especially important if you are trying to reduce sugar intake.

You need to become more mindful of what you are putting into your body with each bite you take. You cannot afford to be ignorant of the amount of sugar (and other fake stuff) is in the foods you eat. Since you are not on Tatooine eating sand for breakfast and rodents for lunch, you have to decide what you eat everyday.

ABC news polled 1000 (http://abcn.ws/2p4Mz2I) people on their breakfast habits. 31% said that they eat cold cereal in the morning.

Now, we can only guess at what kind of cereal they were eating as the poll was not specific in this area, but they were probably eating something more like Lucky Charms, Fruit Loops, or Captain Crunch, each of which has around 12 grams of sugar per serving. And let's be honest, no one eats just one serving of cereal, right? That would be as crazy as eating only one piece of chocolate!

These sugary cereals are part of a complete breakfast, according to what certain brands have led us to believe. Can you picture the standard cereal commercial in your mind's eye? As they say "part of a complete breakfast," you see a glass of milk, a glass of orange juice, a piece of fruit, and a full bowl of dessert.

I grew up on these cereals, and I grew up believing these lies because I had nothing else to go on. I ate cereal every day. I ate cereal at least twice a day. I was oblivious to my sugar intake and oblivious to the fact that sugar was terrible for me. There just wasn't anything out there to tell me otherwise.

Now is the time to become mindful and recognize what is going into your body. It doesn't matter if you are 12 or 68; you have the opportunity to recognize foods for what they are.

I can't possibly list every single food and its sugar content, but will run through some of the most common everyday food items people eat that are surprisingly high in sugar, along with an alternative option for you to consider. Replacing these high-sugar foods is a great first step in defeating the sugar beast.

I strongly suggest getting an app like Fooducate to learn more about foods. You need to start learning about those specific foods that you're eating every day. I am not endorsing the grades that fooducate gives to foods as the end all, be all of food coding, but the information can be really helpful. It can be really hard to read a food label these days despite our best attempts to learn how to do so.

Here are 10 foods you definitely want to avoid to reduce sugar intake. Included with each are some alternative options that are much lower in sugar content:

One: High-Sugar Breakfast Cereals

I mentioned breakfast cereals above because they are an immensely popular food. However, the sugar content is so high that most of these cereals are a terrible choice to start your day. Anything above 10 grams of sugar per serving is a no go. You want to shoot for 5 grams or less.

If you want to eat cereal every day, go for corn flakes, bran flakes, or check out these other high fiber cereals (http://bit.ly/2oECBZV) from Fiber Guardian.com. My blog post goes in depth about which cereals are best for you. It is currently the #1 post on the internet about cereals and hangs around the top 3 on google when searching for "high fiber cereals."

Gloating aside, it is a good resource if you love cereals like I do but also want to start off the day right.

Two: Sauces

If you're like me, you LOVE sauces. You love pouring BBQ sauce over your grilled chicken before AND after you cook it. The tangy, sweet, and savory taste will cause you to salivate just reading about it. BBQ sauce is so delicious, is it any wonder that it's full of sugar?

For example, Kraft Hickory Smoke BBQ sauce has 9 grams of sugar per serving, and a serving size is 2 Tbsp.

And this sauce (as well as other sauces) has high fructose corn syrup, which we know is bad. Considering an average BBQ chicken wing is covered with at least ½ a serving of sauce, we can get a surprising amount of our daily sugar from this kind of food.

Along with bbq sauce; cranberry sauce, relish, spaghetti sauce and yes, even the beloved ketchup are high in sugar.

I love ketchup and it's hard for me to write those words. I've always loved it. A familiar story often told around the Ring household was one that had me sitting in Fenway Park in Boston. In my hands was a seemingly innocent bucket of fries doused in ketchup.

In my defense, I was unable to procure a small cup to carry a side of ketchup in, so I did the next best thing a 10 year old could think of- I covered my fries in ketchup to make sure that I had enough for the journey into the bleacher seats.

To this day, 17 years later, I still get made fun of, and I still love ketchup just as much. It is super hard for me to say no to a side of fries with extra ketchup, even though I know that's a terrible decision for multiple reasons.

The struggle is real. I am right there with you.

Three: Fruit Juice

Say goodbye to apple juice, orange juice, and cranberry juice if you want to reduce your sugar intake. Some of these juices have almost as much (or more sometimes) sugar as soda, and soda is enemy #1.

The best alternative to drinking fruit juice is the obvious one: eat more fruit instead. Juicy pineapple, strawberries, or an orange are just as tasty if you don't pour them in your glass.

Try keeping apples in the fridge. This makes them extra juicy and they will taste extra sweet.

Another good alternative is to make a fruit smoothie. Depending on how you make them, smoothies can be really high in sugar, but that is okay if most of that sugar is not of the "added" variety since that is what we are trying to avoid. Don't hide 4 Tbsp of honey in the smoothie okay?

My current favorite smoothie recipe is as follows. Almost anything that you make from scratch is going to be better than a processed smoothie you might buy, such as the Naked brand which has more sugar than soda and scores a C- on Fooducate…

Banana- bananas are high in fiber, potassium, and are just ridiculously good for you.

Kefir- A splash to give the smoothie a smooth yogurt taste as well as a probiotic boost.

Unsweetened Coconut Milk- Coconut milk is low in sugar and gives the smoothie a liquid base.

Frozen berries, mangoes, pineapples, etc. Berries are super high in antioxidants and are the definition of a superfood.

A spoonful of protein powder to up the protein content. Recommended if you usually drink a smoothie after a workout, like I do.

Honey- I add honey because it is a natural decongestant which helps with my allergies. Make sure it is the raw variety!

This smoothie tastes fabulous, gives you a solid energy boost, and you can be confident that it is healthy for you. It may be high in sugar because of the fruit, but the more fruit the better, just don't have a smoothie for every meal of the day.

Four: Chocolate Milk

Milk in and of itself is a healthy drink due to its high protein, fat, and calcium content; sweetened chocolate milk is a different story. Chocolate milk can still make for a great post-workout recovery drink, but it should be drunk only sparingly. The sugar in it is added and this should be avoided at all costs!

As alternative option and If you are feeling adventurous you can make your own (http://bit.ly/2p51Xwc) healthier version of chocolate milk. Again, don't drink too much--no more than <1, 2> servings. Remember that anything with too much added sugar should be avoided. If you like regular milk, stick with that and avoid the chocolate option.

Five: Granola

Granola is another one of those "health foods" that people want to believe is good for them. However, it's usually high in sugar, and not that high in fiber or protein.

Granola bars are the same story here. They are not a great option for breakfast. Try adding granola to some berries or yogurt to make a more well-rounded meal.

The best option is to pick another high-fiber breakfast option instead of granola. It can be cereal if you want, or a type of granola that is mixed with nuts or another type of health food. Granola on its own isn't anything special.

Six: Sweetened Iced Tea

Once again we face the problem of added sugar. Sweetened iced tea is the definition of added sugar. Take something that is actually healthy for you (regular unsweetened tea), add sugar to it, and what happens? It's no longer good for you at all. Sugar kills all attempts at making something healthy.

The sugar beast loves this type of drink, because it seems so innocent. Surely I can't be doing my body too much harm from a small glass of tea? Except one glass of tea contains almost a full day's worth of sugar.

The best alternative is to drink water with lemon, or have unsweetened tea with a lemon added. Lemons aid in digestive health and add a refreshing taste to the drink without adding any sugar. You are better off avoiding tea completely if you can't have it without a little boost of the white stuff.

Seven: Protein Bars, Granola Bars, and Fiber Bars

Nutritional bars are not created equally. Not at all. There are so many "healthy" food bars out there nowadays that one could have an entire diet based solely off of eating them! Not that you'd want to do that, but the option would be there.

What so-called health food bars come to mind? Clif, Kind, Power, or Nature Valley are just a few popular brands, but taking a stroll down the cereal aisle will give you many more options to choose from.

It's probably best to avoid bars in general since there can be many unknown ingredients within the food. Even Kind bars, which I love, don't get a very high score on fooducate (C+) due to hidden sugars. The Caramel Almond and Sea Salt variety only has 5 grams of sugar listed, which sounds good...until you read that it lists other fake sugars on the ingredient list. This was news to me as of writing this book, and I found it to be disheartening but also enlightening. I now have to avoid eating these bars as well as I don't want to introduce any type of fake sugar into my bloodstream.

This has happened to me several times over the course over the last few years. I find a food that I really like and eat it, thinking that it is good for me. True, eating a Kind bar is better than eating an Egg McMuffin, but it wasn't the best choice. I needed to continue to upgrade my eating habits and strive for the best.

Continuous upgrades over time are the key to long-term success of any kind.

In this case, if I choose to eat a bar, I need to choose a more natural type that is low in sugar of any type and high in protein and fiber. I would recommend either Nugo Fiber Bars or a brand called Oatmega. Both of these brands rate better on Fooducate and they taste great too.

Eight: Vitamin Water, Gatorade, Powerade

One thing these drinks all have in common? Yup, added sugar.

Once again, the health food market ignores the fact that sugar is bad for you and pushes these drinks onto the general population. I am extremely guilty of drinking Gatorade to replenish my lost electrolytes during a workout because it seemed like the right thing to do. I didn't know that Gatorade was terrible for you, and that is has a D+ rating on Fooducate.

As Steve Kamb from Nerd Fitness discusses in his post on the subject (http://bit.ly/2nHtcvs), Gatorade is great if you are doing multiple hours of high intensity physical activity such as running a marathon or playing in an Ultimate Frisbee championship, because it will hydrate you faster than plain water. For anything else, water is just fine.

If you are hitting the gym for 45 minutes to lose weight, chugging a sugary bottle of Gatorade during the workout will erase some of the gains you just realized.

If you are a marathon runner, olympic gymnast, or a regular attendee at the Tour De France, you can choose Gatorade for your hydration needs, but anyone else should avoid it at all costs.

Nine: Canned Fruit

Fruit is good for you. This is true, but you need to be aware that canned fruit is not the same thing. Most canned fruit is stored and preserved in a sugary syrup and stripped of its skin, which reduces fiber content.

Go for natural fruit and avoid those packed into a tiny can.

Ten: Baked Beans

Beans (legumes) are some of the best foods you can eat for losing weight and being healthy. They are high in fiber and protein and taste great too.

However, the baked bean variety is often highly processed and includes a lot of sodium and sugar. If you're looking to add beans into your diet, choose another option such as navy, kidney, or pinto beans. You can make a fantastic chili with beans and it can be one of the best foods for you.

Here is my classic chili recipe (http://bit.ly/2oEMIxO) that I ate quite often in order to lose over 50 pounds after I finished college. I cook the recipe in a slow cooker, but you can cook it quickly over a stovetop if you prefer.

Hopefully this list puts you on the right track to becoming more mindful of the food you choose to feed yourself with. It isn't easy to come to terms with a lot of this stuff right away, especially if you have a lot of bad habits.

Give yourself time and make as many good decisions as you can each and every day. Be aware of what you are putting into your body and become one with the force. You will be a Jedi master soon, young padawan; patience is all you need.

Chapter Six:
Choosing the Right Foods

After learning about the constant deluge of sugar we're putting into our bodies, where do we turn next? Sure, we now have a few alternatives to some of the really bad foods, but what should we eat for breakfast, lunch, and dinner? What should we eat when all we have in the fridge is half a birthday cake?

This was the most difficult thing that I had to deal with when I wanted to lose weight. I struggled with the how, especially when it came to foods. I knew the basics of lifting weights, how to run, and other exercise fundamentals. What I didn't know was anything to do with nutrition and how to eat right.

Fast forward to today and I know slightly more than I did then. I know that there are so many different kinds of foods out there, and so many healthy ones.

It's truly enlightening to know how many good foods exist for us to eat, provided that we can find them. We do not have to feel relegated to just eating burgers, fries, chicken wings, and chocolate shakes.

Eating the right foods satisfies our bodies and will be the #1 way to find peace with sweets. If our bodies are satisfied then we won't feel the extreme urge to eat dessert or desperately try to remember where we hid that last Snickers Bar.

My suggested game plan for a healthy diet is to keep it as simple as possible. The food should be:

1. High in fiber
2. high in protein
3. Low in added sugar

When you are starting out, everything else after this is just another thing to look at.

Of course you are better off looking at every aspect of every food that you eat, but that isn't realistic, at least at first. For the purpose of finding peace with sweets we can keep it simple to start.

The following ten foods are suggestions that meet each of the requirements above. Remember that while we are trying to keep it simple, a balanced diet is key. Don't go to the extreme and decide that you are going to become a forest dweller and eat nuts for the rest of your life. I guess that's a good way to avoid eating sugar, but do you really wanna miss the next Marvel movie and the Super Bowl?

1) Any Fruit

Fruit is an excellent choice to start out your day, or eat at any time of day. Bananas, apples, and oranges are the more common ones, but fruits like starfruit, peaches, and apricots work great as well. Fruits have no added sugar, (unless you dip them in caramel, but please… HAVE YOU READ ANY OF THIS BOOK YET!?) and they are high in fiber with a small amount of protein too.

Fruit is a fantastic way to achieve the energy boost that your body needs when you start the day.

2) Any Vegetable

There is a good reason why it's common knowledge that you should eat more vegetables. Why then do so many people forgo the multicolored delights at their fingertips?

For me it was because I thought vegetables were gross, so I didn't eat them. Most people that don't eat veggies today probably have similar sentiments. It admittedly took me quite a while to venture beyond a salad covered in Thousand Island dressing to eating steamed broccoli, to eating plain ol' cold broccoli (okay only once in awhile…).

Vegetables are high in fiber, and have no added sugar because they are natural.

I love this comparison (http://bit.ly/1aJhB88) of what 200 calories looks like in different foods. You can eat an entire plate of broccoli and only get a few hundred calories while getting a ton of fiber, vitamins, minerals, and other nutrients.

If you eat veggies you will feel good about yourself. Eating fruits and vegetables gives us the freedom and the peace of mind to make decisions about our food intake without feeling as if some supernatural force is making our hands grab the jar of M&Ms and pour it into our waiting maw.

3) Nuts of any Kind

You could write a book on the health benefits and reasons to eat nuts such as almonds, pistachios, walnuts, chestnuts, and cashews. Nuts are high in fiber, protein, and have only about 1 gram of natural sugar per ounce.

I wish I could make a cool analogy that talks about the relationship between nuts and how smart squirrels are, but since squirrels are probably one of the dumbest animals in existence, it's impossible to do so. However, even though nuts don't seem to help out the brains of squirrels very much, we know they do us a lot of good.

This list (http://bit.ly/1sosZtz) is a more comprehensive look at the benefits of eating almonds in particular. Suffice it to say that I personally can't wait to start eating more of any type of nut.

4) Oatmeal

As long as you find the right recipe and the right kind of oatmeal, you will probably want to eat it every day. I suggest cooking up a large batch at the beginning of the week and eat it for breakfast throughout the week.

There are several different varieties, so be mindful that some are loaded with sugar. It can be okay to add a small spoonful of brown sugar if you need to for the taste, just remember that brown sugar counts as added sugar.

5) Avocado Toast

This is a combination of foods, but it makes for an interesting idea. Here is the recipe (http://bit.ly/2nfTOsm), but basically you mash up an avocado, and spread it over wheat toast as a jam. It makes for a really high fiber breakfast.

Avocados are one of those superfoods that are extremely good for you for many different reasons. Adding them to your diet on occasion is a great choice and I will be really freaking proud of you.

6) Fish

The best kind of fish to eat is arguably salmon, but most types of fish are going to be high in protein. Fish have no fiber, but they don't have any sugars either.

Fish are high in Omega-3 fatty acids which promote heart health and are great for weight loss. Eating fish will also help to curb the rush and desire to eat sugar because your body will be pleased by the nutrients it's getting.

Think of your body like an angry child that didn't get what he wanted for Christmas. Just like the child would whine, complain and cry until he got something else, your body will never be satisfied by a Burger King Chicken Deluxe. It will keep on asking for more until it can't possibly eat any more.

Instead, give your body what it desires with a meal consisting of fresh baked salmon, steamed asparagus, a small dinner roll, and even a glass of red wine and see if the angry kid comes out then. Hint: he won't, because his Christmas was freaking awesome. He is happy and satisfied and feeling content.

7) Sweet Potatoes

Sweet potatoes are a perfect alternative low sugar food. They are high in fiber, potassium, and rich in Vitamin A, which can promote a healthy immune system. Most importantly they have only about 5 grams of real sugar.

There are an abundant number of recipes that you

can add sweet potatoes to, but the best way to eat a potato is to either bake or microwave a whole spud and go to town. I eat the skin to be sure to get all of the nutrients and fiber, but even just the mushy part is really good for you.

8) Seeds

If you are a fan of chewing on sunflower seeds when playing a sport then there is good news because that is an excellent habit. Any type of seeds such as pumpkin, sunflower, flax, chia, sesame, etc. are all low sugar and good for you.

Seeds make a great addition to a salad or a smoothie. They are ripe with benefits.

9) Eggs

Don't believe anything you read that says that eggs are unhealthy. While researching this chapter I came across a forum on health boards.com that read- "Eggs are not healthy. The yolk alone is two points on WW (Weight Watchers)."

Reading stuff like this makes me cringe! Whoever wrote this actually believes it. Can't you just see the sugar beast smiling from his chocolate-covered throne?

Still another found on Yahoo "How many points are diet sodas in Weight Watchers? The answer given- "Diet soda's have a 0 calorie value since you probably burn it off as you drink it."

Ahh! There is so much truth out there that is covered by such nonsense. Calories are not king. The sugar beast is laughing maniacally at that, I am sure.

Just one large egg has 6 grams of protein and a negligible amount of sugar. Eggs are a normal way for a lot of Americans to start their day, and for good reason, as they are packed with nutrients.

There is no wrong way to eat an egg (unless of course you are one of those that just drinks uncooked eggs, blech) but the best way is to boil it. Boiling eggs is probably the easiest way to prepare them, but it is also the most healthy. If you prefer to fry the egg that is okay, but be aware that any time you are frying something in oil or butter you are adding to the natural product.

That being said, eggs of any kind are better than no eggs at all. They will provide you with energy and an excellent alternative to sugar-laden breakfast foods such as donuts.

10) Beans

If baked beans are a food to avoid, the beans of any other kind are to be eaten whenever possible. Beans are super high in protein, super high in fiber, and have zero added sugar.

I get my beans from a can, but you can get fresh beans as well. The salt content on canned beans is high, but I recommend draining them to reduce this.

Beans were the staple of my diet when I was losing weight after college, and I think I owe it to beans to share with the world their transformative powers.

All of these foods are ones that you should eat more of. They will keep you feeling satisfied and full and the sugar beast won't be able to get you as easily.

Better yet, once you start to eat these foods you will begin to crave the energy boost you get when eating nuts, eggs, and fruits. The cravings for unhealthy foods will eventually reduce, and you will be able to actually enjoy a dessert for once, instead of scarfing it down in three seconds flat.

Chapter Seven:
Prep the Battleground

You will find major success by reinventing your health fortress: the foods you surround yourself with and how you spend each day. This progress can happen slowly over time, but even slowly, gradual smart choices will guide you to become the person you want to be.

This holds true in business, personal finance, nutrition, weight loss, relationships, and other areas of life. What you do for a living, how you spend your money, what you put into your body, and who you spend time with all affect you.

This will be the same for reducing sugar intake. If you surround yourself with sugary drinks, sweet snacks, and candy canes, you will be very likely to eat them. If you keep apples, bananas, and oranges lying around, you will probably eat those instead. You cannot argue with this logic, unless of course you don't count "emergency chocolate" as a sugary food.

Wherever you call home, whether it's an apartment, a duplex, or a mansion, you should be aware that it is a battleground. It is THE battleground! In order to fight the war on sugar and defeat the sugar beast you will need to prep your battleground.

All of the great generals in history understood the importance of preparing their battlefields. Whether is was digging trenches, placing sandbags, or setting up communications systems, a war could not be fought without preparation.

Do you think General George Patton would have allowed his troops to lounge around and play volleyball when they could have been placing sandbags and digging trenches? Nope!

Here are seven ways you can prepare the battlefield at home and at work in order to win the war on sugar. Put your armor on and get ready to do battle. The sugar beast will not be happy when he finds out you read and applied this section...

1) Meal Prep

Prepping meals in advance is a new way of getting meals ready for the week. The basic gist involves spending a few hours on a Sunday cooking and prepping meals for the entire week. This way you can bring food to work and have your supper all ready for you when you come home during the workweek.

This time investment early on in the week will save you oodles of time overall. Who doesn't like the idea of sitting down to read a good book instead of cooking supper for a family of four?

You need three things to make this work:

A good set of food storage containers (hint: look online for some great deals).

A variety of healthy recipes (http://bit.ly/1ETdlAb) to choose from. You can create your own or check out some of the ideas from that link. Remember that chili recipe I gave you earlier? You can make that and it will last for about a week for a single person.

A little bit of time to get it together. If you live with other people, bring them into the process. A family that cooks together stays together, or at least, you'll have extra time to watch a movie together during the week.

Prepping meals in advance is like preparing for a week-long hike. You get everything ready in advance because you won't be able to return home for forgotten items. You are stuck with what you brought.

While this same logic won't apply as you drive past the grocery store on your commute back from work, it is helpful to be in this mindset.

Prepare early on and get everything that you will need. This amount of planning might prove difficult at first, but once you bring something that can be heated up while at work, you will feel like a superstar.

A hot, nutritious meal will give you the energy boost you need to get through your day. Your cravings for a donut from the break room will diminish. Why eat a donut when you can have a cup of homemade chili? Your body will thank you.

2) Share the Love

Share with your coworkers and family members that you are trying to reduce your sugar intake. Better yet, gift them a copy of this book and show them what you are working on. (That may have been a shameless plug to sell another book, but you can't blame me for trying to spread the word!)

It can be scary to tell people that you're trying to lose weight and live healthier, because of the real fear that they might judge you. But I think that if you give people the chance, they might surprise you. They may even want to join you in your journey.

It is A LOT harder to eat the last cupcake in the box if you know that other people are aware of your attempt to consume less sugar. It isn't about them judging you or looking down on you; it's about you staying accountable. If others are aware of your goals and are truly your friends, they will want to see you succeed.

Of course, following this line of advice does bring with it some risks. Change can be scary to some people, even change that exists outside themselves. Because we live in a culture that is focused on me me ME, we might resent others for wanting to better themselves.

That being said, involving other people in your goal will make a dramatic difference in your follow through and progress.

3) Gather the Fruits and Veggies

As I have hinted at in earlier chapters, fruits and veggies are the way to go. Captain America wouldn't be complete with Bucky, Han Solo would be in big trouble without Chewy, and Frodo would be pretty lame if not for Samwise. Fruits and veggies are the bane of all snack food companies because they are responsible for lost revenue.

One of the best ways to reduce sugar intake is to have suitable replacements ready and available at the drop of a hat. If you get a sugar craving, grab an apple and go to town. Not only are apples filling and juicy, eating them requires a time commitment. By the time you get to the core your sugar craving should be quite satisfied.

The same goes for most vegetables. Eating a few carrots and celery with a little bit of ranch dressing can be an extremely good snack. With each satisfying snap, any craving you had for a Snickers bar will fade away. It won't completely knock out the craving, especially at first, but it will take the edge off.

Once you start to satisfy sugar cravings with these natural whole foods, you'll start to crave these foods instead. The cravings will be nowhere near as intense as their unnatural counterparts, but things will start to level out. The need for certain foods will become a need of hunger instead of a need so strong you would consider digging for chocolate truffles as a great way to spend an afternoon.

Have fruits and veggies readily available by using a similar tactic to meal prepping. Have bags of carrots, celery, broccoli, or perhaps cauliflower ready to go. You can dip them in a low sugar dipping sauce, just don't go overboard. Keep apples in your fridge and bananas stocked on the counter. Have frozen berries in the freezer to add to smoothies or shakes.

The key is to purposely choose to eat these foods by making them the easy choice. If something filled with addictive sugar is staring you right in the face, there's a good chance you will choose to eat that instead of the natural, healthy options.

We don't have the ability to consistently fight off the desire to say yes to chocolate and sweets. In order to fight back we have to adjust our environment and add the right foods to our pantries and refrigerators.

4) Sleep Enough

If we get enough sleep our body will repair itself overnight. If we skip this process things begin to break down and the battleground can become a dark and scary place.

How many times have you stayed up too late and felt mad sugar cravings the next day? Your body needs energy. If it doesn't get the energy through sleep and natural foods, the brain will trick us into getting the energy another way.

The body says, "Look buddy, I'm going to get what I want regardless of how you give it to me."

When levels of sleep go down, energy stores dwindle. We then try to replace the energy lost with foods that give us a rapid energy boost. Our brains are wired to know that the energy released from those foods will be quick and pleasing to us in the short term.

The problem is that we are wired for this short term survival instinct because our prehistoric ancestors did not have to worry about these types of foods. Instead they had to worry about being run down by a herd of rams or being eaten alive. There was no fear of a slow death by processed foods.

As it pertains to our health and war against sugar, we need to focus on getting enough sleep as a primary battle tactic. The times we live in are different and therefore we must continue to adapt.

5) Drink Enough Water

You might be thinking, "Enough already! I know I should drink water, stop telling me!"

My answer is no, I won't stop telling you. It saddens me how many people won't drink water because they don't like the taste. Your body likes water and what it does for you so drink up.

But, why is water important to your health and well being? Keeping your body hydrated has quite a few amazing benefits, including keeping you energized and awake, and allowing you to stay focused. Water also helps to maintain normal bowel function.

Most importantly to our topic here, is that hunger

and cravings often arise when we are dehydrated. We can stay ahead of sugar cravings and fake hunger if we stay hydrated.

If you don't often feel thirsty AND you don't drink water on a regular basis this could be a sign that your thirst mechanism is out of balance. This balance problem is caused by reaching for alternatives other than water to quench your thirst.

For a healthy person a good sign that they need to drink more water is the feeling of thirst. For many, this process gets broken down over time when we become accustomed to a sedentary lifestyle and sugary foods. To reverse this we cannot wait for our bodies to tell us that we are thirsty, we must stay ahead of the game.

For those that struggle to drink water, you are certainly not alone. I grew up not drinking water. My liquid intake was mostly juice, soda, and ice tea. I never really liked the taste of water and I refused to drink it regularly. My thirst mechanism was way out of sync and I was chronically dehydrated.

It wasn't until I met my wife and became accustomed to her water-drinking habits that I truly found the benefits of staying hydrated.

Drinking more water is as simple as having a glass when you wake up, drinking a glass before each meal, and drinking water instead of snacking in the afternoon. You can also add lemon to your water for additional flavor, invest in a quality water filter, or eat water packed foods like fruit.

Regardless of which way will work for you, drinking more water and having more of it around is a must to defeat the sugar beast!

6) Treat Yo Self

The fantastic news about peace with sweets means you can have sweet food every once in awhile. We're not talking about a complete denial of the foods we love. Your older sibling is not waving a finger at you, forbidding you to ever again ride her bicycle.

Once you get your cravings under control, don't be afraid to eat a piece of red velvet cake every once in awhile. The idea is just to enjoy these foods and be able to move on. We do not want to eat one and then think about eating the next one right after we put the fork down.

We must be able to put down the fork, be thankful that God blessed the world with such sweet delectable items, and forgo third or fourth helpings.

Treat yourself every once in awhile by having small chocolates or candies around the house. They key is to keep them small in order to not undo the progress you are making.

7) Quit Cold Turkey

If none of the other methods work for you over the long term, you might have to go cold turkey. This means a complete abstinence from eating any added sugars. For me, it wouldn't mean staying away from any type of sugar, because that isn't good for you. What it does mean is no real "sweets" of any kind.

Take a few weeks and get it completely out of your system. After that, figure out how you feel and go from there. If you can reasonably start adding sweets into your diet and not lose control, then by all means do so. If eating one chocolate bar sets you over the deep end, then for you, "peace with sweets" might not be possible after a month.

For most extreme cases of sugar addiction, a time away from added sugar could be just the change that you need.

Altering the battlefield involves having the right mindset for success. If you are able to incorporate these six (or all seven if needed!) strategies into your campaign to destroy the sugar beast, you will at last be able to come to peace with sweets.

Chapter Eight: Exercise as a Means Of Reducing Cravings

I am a huge fan of exercise as a remedy for all kinds of problems.

Feel bad? Go for a run.

Feel stressed? Do a yoga session.

Feel tired? Lift some weights.

Feel depressed? Go for a short walk around the neighborhood.

Along with all of these other benefits, exercise in any form can reduce sugar cravings. How does it do this?

For one, it gives you some distance from the craving. If you are on a run, the last thing you want to do during the run is to snack on a brownie. You will be outside in the sunshine (or inside running on a treadmill watching Discovery Channel) and you will not have access to any sweets.

Secondly, doing any kind of exercise releases endorphins. These little neurotransmitters are chemicals that pass along signals from one neuron to the next in your nervous system. When you do a physical activity like running, endorphins are released in your system and create a feeling of pleasure similar to the feeling the drug morphine induces.

Doing something active of any kind is a fantastic way to reduce cravings, because it gives you something else to do other than sit there and think about the chocolate cake your boss just brought over. It also releases other chemicals in your body such as the endorphins that take the place of the feeling you were hoping to get from the sugary snack.

Even getting out of your desk chair and doing a few tricep dips can swing your thoughts and desires in the right direction. The thoughts become "Oh man, my triceps are legit," instead of "How can I rationalize eating this cake?" (Which is usually said in your head DUR-

ING the cake consumption.)

If you're trying to win the war on sugar, you can't do so if you get into a staring match with a Krispy Kreme donut. You will lose every single time. Donuts are known for their wildly overpowering mind tricks. They send out thoughts like "beam me up Scotty." Yet instead of Captain Kirk materializing aboard the enterprise the donut smiles as it enters your gullet.

The battle is so difficult to win that we need an outlet for our desires that goes beyond food replacement. The good news is that there are so many ways to stay active and exercise that no one has a good excuse not to do so. There are literally hundreds of activities that you could get into right away to up your endorphin level, reduce sugar cravings, and of course get to your ideal weight.

Here are just a few that I recommend that are fun and sure to get you feeling good:

Walking – Start walking everywhere that you can! Walking can be a lot of fun, especially if you're into audiobooks like I am. I love to take a stroll and listen to a good book, especially when the weather is nice.

Running -- This is a step up from walking, but it is one of the best exercises in terms of getting a full body workout. Running is also one of the best ways to feel the "runner's high" or the feeling of endorphins flooding into your system.

HIIT -- HIIT stands for high intensity interval training. You can do intervals with any sport or activity but it involves alternating bursts of high intensity workout sessions with breaks in between. HIIT is especially effective because it takes less time and does more than walking or running.

Tennis – Tennis is a lifelong sport that only takes a court, a few balls, a racket, and a friend. Or better yet, make it a party and get three other people involved! Tennis is a good example of a sport that can be related to interval training, as you are mixing in high intensity rallies with rest periods in between to switch sides and to serve.

Racquetball – Sets can be found at many gyms, and it's a great workout. The first time I played, I felt like I was going to die from working so hard. It is an extreme way to get a solid workout in while having fun.

Ping Pong – Ping Pong may not seem like much, but if you get into it, you'll find yourself sweating shortly into playing.

Volleyball – It's a great team sport for having fun. Do 2v2 or 3v3 for the best physical impact.

Swimming – Swimming is one of the best exercises for you, because you don't put as much stress on your joints as you do when running or lifting weights.

Ultimate Frisbee – This is my personal favorite sport ever. It's very similar to soccer in that you spend most of your time running. It's also one of the best sports for burning calories!

Disc golf – It's not as intense as ultimate frisbee, but you do get a lot of walking in when playing this sport.

Hiking – Hiking is a great way to enjoy nature and get a workout in all at the same time. My wife and I absolutely love hiking, and have dedicated an entire website (http://www.twohikershiking.com) to our adventures. Go ahead and check it out to get motivated!

Surfing – I've never surfed, but if you're near a beach, why not try this out?

Parkour – I would be too scared of breaking bones, but doing parkour or freerunning is a great way to stay active.

Dancing – Just dancing around the house is good enough for this one, but you can indeed get into dance as a hobby too!

Gardening – Yes gardening is a great hobby to get into and a great way to shed off some extra pounds.

Kickball – I think kickball is super boring, but I have a lot of friends that love it for some reason I will never understand. But that's just my opinion. Don't knock it until you try it!

Any league sport, such as soccer, flag football, or basketball. Competition brings out an extra level of exertion all while having a good time.

There are so many more sports and hobbies that you can get into that are both physical and fun that this list could span an entire book. For now, try and get involved in some sort of hobby that involves exercise. This will lead you to feel better about yourself and will just be another part of the fantastic new life you are building for yourself.

Every time you swing that racket and hit a tennis ball, the sugar beast cries. He weeps for a lost subject and lost chance to claim another victim.

Chapter Nine: Build Your Personal Blueprint

In order to ultimately vanquish the sugar beast and find peace with sweets, you need to build a blueprint. This means coming up with a gameplan that works for you. This means putting together all that you have learned so far in reading this book and formulating a battle plan.

Merriam Webster defines "blueprint" as a "detailed plan or program of action."

Your personal blueprint to reduce sugar intake needs to consist of a detailed plan with plenty of action steps to act upon that plan. Creating this blueprint requires you to take the advice I've written here and organize it into manageable bite size pieces.

The only real shot you have to reach your goals is to do it your own unique way. We were all created with different abilities, as well as different likes and dislikes. While I am not overly fond of swimming, you might be a dolphin. You might be someone that enjoys eating nuts all day, but hates the taste of any type of fruit.

With that in mind, ask yourself the following questions. They will help you build your own blueprint for reducing sugar intake. I will also share several samples of what a blueprint might look like.

What Medium do You Prefer?

The first step in creating your own personal blueprint is to decide on the medium for that blueprint. It doesn't have to be a thin, blue and white piece of paper that you carry around. It can actually be whatever you would like.

I personally love white boards and keeping track of goals via this method. The reason? Because they are big and right in your face. I walk by the boards multiple times per day and am forced to see what I'm working on. My friends make fun of me for my "goal boards," but I don't care. I enjoy having a direction and a reminder of what I am ultimately working on.

When we have goals that force us to reduce our sugar intake, such as no dessert for two weeks, we're forced to work hard to reach those goals. For me, keeping track in a loud and in-your-face kind of way does wonders for sticking to my blueprint.

Below you will see a picture of my personal goal board that I use to keep track of my progress. My wife and I currently use a version of a goal board that we created after reading Level Up Your Life by Steve Kamb from NerdFitness.com. This is a general goal board not specifically designed to reduce our sugar intake, but to push ourselves and grow in many other ways as well.

If you look closely though, you can see that we had several goals such as "no dessert for two weeks" that really stretched us by reducing our dependence on sugar.

We love it because it is a fantastic way to stay motivated and to keep each other accountable.

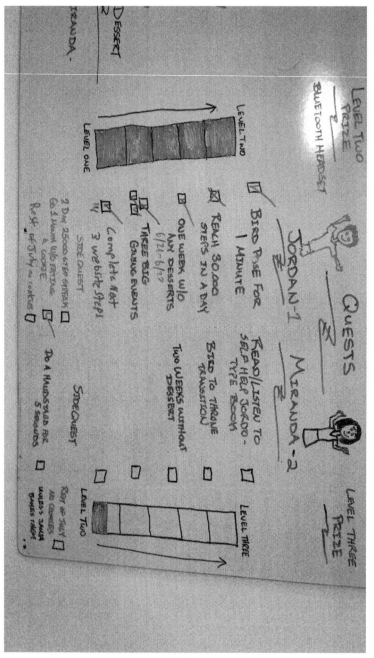

If you aren't a huge fan of white boards then a goal board won't work for you. there are many other options too:

Keep a journal (digital or hardcopy). I keep my journal as a shortcut on my web browser.

Use a Google or Excel spreadsheet. I track everything related to my books and websites in one giant spreadsheet. It's as literally awesome as you can metaphorically get.

Carry a small postcard with your goals written down in a succinct way. I have never tried this, but I think it could be seriously helpful to carry along a constant reminder. It could even be something you attach to your key ring, such as a reminder to "not feed the beast!"

Make a one page hard copy that you can print out and keep with you. Print it on cardstock to give it a little extra feeling of importance.

Utilize an online service such as Lifetick to set and track goals via an app.

For recording your blueprint, use anything works that works for you. Nothing you do will work if it doesn't align with your lifestyle and your goals. The next big fad diet to reduce sugar intake will not work for you unless you can find a way to incorporate it into your life.

What Do You Struggle With the Most?

In a way, I'm uniquely qualified to write this book, because the struggle with the sugar monster is all too real. I'm someone who loves sweets and will never easily pass up on freshly baked cookies.

Cookies are my kryptonite. My wife and I have this in common. If one of us wants to break from the plan and eat a cookie, the other is ecstatic because it means that they too can eat a cookie (or two or five…).

Your personal blueprint needs to have a part that mentions your weakness and your plan to defeat it. If you love brownies, limit yourself to one per week by buying just one from a local bakery. It will taste amazing and it won't upset your goals. If you are really brave, eat just one per month (ouch, stop holding this book so tight!).

If you salivate when even thinking about milkshakes, make them homemade to limit added sugar and other ingredients. If you must start out the day with a coffee and a donut, at least don't add sugar to your coffee. If you love cookies, make protein cookies or quit cold turkey like my wife and I had to.

We were eating so many cookies that we had to quit for 2 months just to not have three or more a day. When there's a chef making cookies daily at your day job, it's REALLY hard not to eat them, especially when we're tasked with putting said cookies in the grab and go bin for our residents.

A lot of your biggest struggles can be minimized by being in control of the ingredients and making things homemade, but sometimes you might just have to quit cold turkey.

How you overcome your biggest weakness is up to you, but do so and you will be that much closer to finding peace with sweets and locking up the sugar beast for good.

What's the Point?

The rest of the blueprint should focus on the part of your struggle that needs the most improvement.

To come up with ideas you can make a bullet list or make up some funny phrases to keep it interesting such as "stop eating cookies jerkface," "Did you eat your veggies today big guy?," or even "Hey girl, no shakes for you this week!"

Is there a main area of your battle against sugar that you need to work on? For my wife and I, it is learning to not eat so many cookies. For you, it might be to stop drinking soda or sweet tea. What does your focus need to be? Chances are that you know the answer to that question, you just might not like what you need to do about it.

There needs to be an end goal. Why are you reducing sugar intake and eating all of these freaking veggies? It can't be as boring and unspecific as "I want to feel better."

The goal on your blueprint needs to have a clear and concise direction. Here are a few that will work:

1. I want to up my intake of fruits and veggies and reduce added sugar intake.
2. I want to lose 50 pounds by the end of the year.
3. I want to avoid type 2 diabetes by changing my eating habits.

I don't think it necessarily has to be a goal that you can measure and track relentlessly, because that can be easy to forget to do or might become tedious over time. It just needs to give you a sense of direction.

What Action Steps are You Going to Take?

Now that you have your medium picked out, know your weaknesses and have a clear and concise goal, what are you going to change?

Unfortunately, to reach any actual success with a goal, change must occur. If I am going to stop eating so many cookies I need to set limits and eat less cookies, or better yet, eat no cookies at all.

Similar to our goal board I shared earlier the blueprint needs to have clear and concise action steps, just like:

I won't eat cookies for a month

Drink soda only on Fridays during April

Before each main meal for the next 3 weeks I will drink a full glass of water

I will only have one dessert per day for the next month

What do all of these steps have in common? They are actionable AND will make a difference in your war on sugar. They also force you to become more aware of your surroundings and make important choices based on your long-term desires vs your short-term cravings.

How Badly do You Want it?

This is a question you need to ask yourself in order to continue working on your blueprint. It will shape the final product in a way that will keep you motivated.

How badly do you want to reach your goals and become a healthier, more well-rounded person? I believe that we always should be working to improve ourselves in order to become the best person possible. Are you willing to work crazy hard to reach your ultimate potential?

It can help to add a motivational phrase at the end of the blueprint, a picture of a ripped guy or gal, or even a quote from your favorite author.

In summary the blueprint needs to have:

1. Your choice of medium (whiteboard, postcard, paper, etc.)
2. Your biggest struggles and weaknesses
3. A clear goal
4. Clear action steps to reach that goal
5. A motivational Phrase to help you keep going

Here is an example of a blueprint my wife created for reducing sugar intake:

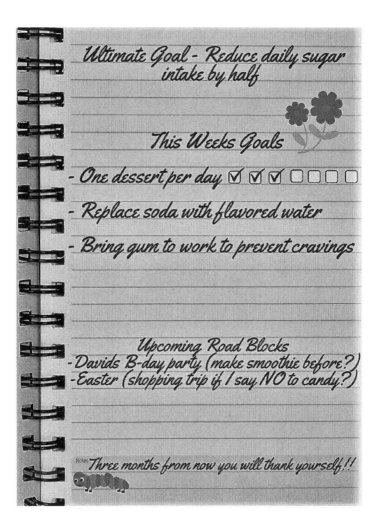

Once you add all of these elements together you will have a fine tuned and personally created tool that will aid you in battle. It will be the shield to use against the forces of evil and you can use it to prevent the sugar beast from throwing cookies at you and begging you to eat them.

You will be at peace knowing that you have a tool ready to use at any time, and will be armed with the knowledge that you are making progress in your goals. There's nothing that will give you more peace and contentment than a winning day.

Chapter Ten: Consistency Through Course Adjustments

Take a glance at this unforgettable dialogue in one of my favorite movies of all time--Star Wars, Revenge of the Sith:

Anakin Skywalker to Obi-Wan Kenobi: Don't make me kill you.
Obi-Wan Kenobi: Anakin, my allegiance is to the Republic, to democracy.
Anakin Skywalker: If you're not with me, then you're my enemy.
Obi-Wan Kenobi: [realizing that Anakin is consumed by evil and there's no reasoning with him anymore] Only a Sith deals in absolutes. I will do what I must.
Anakin Skywalker: You will try.

It was never Obi-Wan Kenobi's intention to do battle with the man he viewed as his brother and best friend. Obi-Wan never wanted to fight Anakin, but for the good of the galaxy he adjusted course. He realized that Anakin was beyond reason and had fully (okay not fully you Star Wars fans!) given himself over to the dark side.

As Obi-Wan drew his lightsaber, he knew he would either be cut down by his friend or strike the final blow himself.

Just like Obi-Wan, we will need to adjust course on the fly in order to win the war on the sugar beast. Our blueprints will not help us in every circumstance, and we will need to make adjustments.

What will we do if Mom makes a surprise visit and brings triple chunk brownies? What will happen if your friend's "home-cooked meal" turns into pizza and a 6-pack? What can you do about that office party that offers basically every unhealthy food known to man?

Just the other day, I was sitting in the office, when one of my coworkers came in with a cupcake specifically for me. It was store bought, surely filled with preservatives, and loaded with sugar, but I ate it because "it was the right thing to do."

It can be hard enough preparing our own battlefield,

but there will ALWAYS be unforeseen and unexpected hiccups in our journey. We have to learn to adjust course and realign our expectations with the new reality.

The challenges you created for yourself a month ago might not be good enough today, nor relevant. You may have started slow by avoiding sugar completely for one day of the week. A month in, you might need to up the ante by going for 2 or 3 days a week.

Sometimes things just aren't working. Sometimes your original plan wasn't good enough and isn't making any noticeable difference. Your progress has stagnated because you aren't doing enough. At this point you must change directions or up the stakes.

In order to stay consistent and actually reach any goal, you need to be willing to adjust course midway through. Even if you set a big goal in the beginning, eventually that big goal will seem pretty small. When you perform beyond your wildest expectations, the only way to keep growing is to increase the challenge or to find a new challenge.

Consistency comes through creating new habits as well as cultivating old ones. When you adjust course and add a level of difficulty, remember to keep doing the stuff that was working for you. If a morning walk keeps you from adding a ton of sugar to your coffee, don't replace the walk with a different activity. Keep doing the things that are working for you and replace or change what isn't working.

Writing a book is a perfect example of the necessity of staying consistent. If I go a week without writing I find it incredibly difficult to jump back into it and to be productive. I spent a whole month "writing" my first book and didn't get anywhere. I knew that if I wanted to finish the book in the time frame that I had set for myself I would need to keep a schedule and write consistently.

I ended up writing over 30,000 words in one month and finished my first book. I adjusted the ship midcourse before I crashed into the iceberg (or in my case, kept pounding my head onto the desk willing the computer to write my book for me). I was able to recognize that I was getting nowhere and needed to make a new game plan.

In the same way you need to see where your blueprint might not be working and adjust accordingly. It may take time and trial and error before you find the mode of operating that works best for you.

All you really need is the willingness to learn and to experience new things. Take it one day at a time and keep fighting. The sugar beast will be defeated, and your ultimate peaceful relationship with sweet treats will ensue.

Final Thoughts and a Kick in the Butt

Discovering a place where you can have a healthy relationship with sweet snacks and sugary drinks doesn't happen overnight. You know that fighting off sugar cravings and reducing sugar intake is hard. You probably got this book hoping that it will make you stronger and better equipped to ward off these cravings and make the need for the sugary intoxication go away.

While I believe in the methods I shared here, you are the captain of your own destiny. You are the one steering the ship. You are in control of your choices and you are ultimately responsible for your fate. Once you fully grasp that you are where you are based on the choices you've made, you'll begin to feel empowered to make a change. Nothing will get in your way.

Defeating the sugar beast is a long-term battle that you will fight for the rest of your life. Do yourself a favor and start the fight now. Start saying no to added sugar and frosted cupcakes. Start stringing together days where you don't eat any added sugar. Start making the change that you know you deserve.

Once you start, the wins will start to come and they will feel amazing. From looking great in the mirror, to the disappearance of cravings, to the ability to say no at any time to any sweet, to the newfound power to eat a piece of cake and enjoy it 100% guilt free.

All of these things can be achieved by you, but the secret lies within.

You are amazing and loved and incredible. Never sell yourself short. ALWAYS believe in yourself. You are uniquely perfect in the eyes of your creator and if we ever get the chance to meet I will tell you that to your face.

I truly believe that everyone in this world has unlimited potential. If we can tap into that potential, together we can rule the galaxy. Or wait, sorry, the Star Wars references came back!

Together we can change the world brick by brick, person by person.

Are you ready to change the world?

A Quick Favor Please?

I sincerely hope that you enjoyed reading this book. I spent a lot of time writing, editing, and researching in order to give you the absolute best product that I can.

I also enjoyed adding in nerdy references when I could. I hope you enjoyed these. If not, forgive my childish sense of humor.

If you ultimately found the book uplifting, insightful, and practically useful, I would appreciate a review. You can click on the link below to be sent right to Amazon in order to rate it. I thank you in advance for doing this.

Every review counts and each one will help others to find the book and to benefit from the words contained within.

Go here to review this book (http://bit.ly/2nO3shW)

-Jordan

About the Author

Jordan Ring is the owner and creator of Fiberguardian.com, TwoHikersHiking.com, and his site dedicated to his writing JMRing.com.

He enjoys making weird faces, doing ridiculous Fiber Guardian videos, eating apples, and playing ultimate frisbee with his wife. He believes in taking action and taking accountability for his own choices, and has made it a life goal to share his ideas with the world.

As of this writing he is an assistant manager at a retirement community and loves making a positive impact on the lives of the residents there. He works with his wife, and enjoys every minute spent with his soul mate.

You can find him by emailing Jordan@jmring.com or by tweeting @AuthorJMRing. He is always available and ready to answer any questions and respond to comments.

Manufactured by Amazon.ca
Bolton, ON